SEX COUPONS FOR

Him

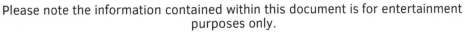

THIS COUPON ENTITLES YOU TO:

A NUDE DINNER SERVICE

0 123456789 87

TERMS & CONDITIONS:

_____

_____

_____

THIS COUPON ENTITLES YOU TO:

A NAKED GAME OF TWISTER, POKER ETC.

0 123456789 87

TERMS & CONDITIONS:
_____

_____

_____

THIS COUPON ENTITLES YOU TO:

THE KINKIEST SEX YOU WANT

0 123456789 87

TERMS & CONDITIONS: _____

_____

_____

THIS COUPON ENTITLES YOU TO:

ONE NIGHT OF VOYERISM

TERMS & CONDITIONS:

0 123456789 87

THIS COUPON ENTITLES YOU TO:

WHOLE BODY KISSING

TERMS & CONDITIONS:

_____

_____

_____

0 123456789 87

THIS COUPON ENTITLES YOU TO:

A FREE NAUGHTY WISH

0 123456789 87

TERMS & CONDITIONS:

_____

_____

_____

THIS COUPON ENTITLES YOU TO:

QUICKIE

TERMS & CONDITIONS:

_____

_____

_____

0 123456789 87

THIS COUPON ENTITLES YOU TO:

A SHOWER FOR TWO

TERMS & CONDITIONS:

_____

_____

_____

0 123456789 87

THIS COUPON ENTITLES YOU TO:

ORAL PLEASURE

0 123456789 87

TERMS & CONDITIONS:

_____

_____

_____

THIS COUPON ENTITLES YOU TO:

NIGHT OF LOVE

TERMS & CONDITIONS:

_____

_____

_____

0 123456789 87

THIS COUPON ENTITLES YOU TO:

A MASSAGE WITH HAPPY ENDING

0 123456789 87

TERMS & CONDITIONS:

_____

_____

_____

THIS COUPON ENTITLES YOU TO:

A YOU-CHOOSE-THE-TOY NIGHT

TERMS & CONDITIONS: _____

_____

_____

0 123456789 87

THIS COUPON ENTITLES YOU TO:

ROLE PLAYING

TERMS & CONDITIONS:

_____

_____

_____

0 123456789 87

THIS COUPON ENTITLES YOU TO:

MIDDLE OF NIGHT SEX

TERMS & CONDITIONS:

0 123456789 87

THIS COUPON ENTITLES YOU TO:

STEAK AND BLOWJOB

TERMS & CONDITIONS:

_____

_____

_____

0 123456789 87

THIS COUPON ENTITLES YOU TO:

A SECRET DESIRE

0 123456789 87

TERMS & CONDITIONS:
_____

_____

_____

THIS COUPON ENTITLES YOU TO:

PLAY DRESS UP

TERMS & CONDITIONS:

_____

_____

_____

0 123456789 87

THIS COUPON ENTITLES YOU TO:

A PASSIONATE EVENING

0 123456789 87

TERMS & CONDITIONS:

_____

_____

_____

THIS COUPON ENTITLES YOU TO:

USE HANDCUFFS

0 123456789 87

TERMS & CONDITIONS:

_____

_____

_____

THIS COUPON ENTITLES YOU TO:

A LONG FOREPLAY

0 123456789 87

TERMS & CONDITIONS:

_____

_____

_____

THIS COUPON ENTITLES YOU TO:

ONE SEX SESSION, ANYTIME, ANYWHERE

TERMS & CONDITIONS: _____

_____

_____

0 123456789 87

THIS COUPON ENTITLES YOU TO:

I'LL TAKE ALL MY CLOTHES OFF, WHATEVER I'M DOING

TERMS & CONDITIONS: _____

_____

_____

0 123456789 87

THIS COUPON ENTITLES YOU TO:

ONE STRIPTEASE

0 123456789 87

TERMS & CONDITIONS:

_____

_____

_____

THIS COUPON ENTITLES YOU TO:

A ROMANTIC BUBBLE BATH FOR TWO

TERMS & CONDITIONS:

0 123456789 87

THIS COUPON ENTITLES YOU TO:

GO SKINNY DIPPING

0 123456789 87

TERMS & CONDITIONS:

_____

_____

_____

THIS COUPON ENTITLES YOU TO:

A NEW SEXY EXPERIMENT

0 123456789 87

TERMS & CONDITIONS:

_____

_____

_____

THIS COUPON ENTITLES YOU TO:

MUSTACHE RIDE

TERMS & CONDITIONS: _____

_____

_____

0 123456789 87

THIS COUPON ENTITLES YOU TO:

TRY ANAL

TERMS & CONDITIONS:

_____

_____

_____

0 123456789 87

THIS COUPON ENTITLES YOU TO:

PLAYTIME IN JUST HEELS

TERMS & CONDITIONS: _____

_____

_____

0 123456789 87

THIS COUPON ENTITLES YOU TO:

MORNING SEX

TERMS & CONDITIONS:

_____

_____

_____

0 123456789 87

THIS COUPON ENTITLES YOU TO:

ONE NEW POSITION EVERY NIGHT FOR A WEEK

TERMS & CONDITIONS:
_____

_____

_____

THIS COUPON ENTITLES YOU TO:

TIE ME UP

TERMS & CONDITIONS:

_____

_____

_____

0 123456789 87

THIS COUPON ENTITLES YOU TO:

15 MINUTES OF BOOBIE TIME

0 123456789 87

TERMS & CONDITIONS:
_____
_____
_____

THIS COUPON ENTITLES YOU TO:

MAKE OUT IN PUBLIC

TERMS & CONDITIONS: _____

_____

_____

0 123456789 87

THIS COUPON ENTITLES YOU TO:

SEX OUTSIDE

TERMS & CONDITIONS: _____

_____

_____

0 123456789 87

THIS COUPON ENTITLES YOU TO:

A HANDJOB

TERMS & CONDITIONS:
_____

_____

_____

0 123456789 87

THIS COUPON ENTITLES YOU TO:

SHE-DOES-ALL-THE-WORK SESSION

TERMS & CONDITIONS:

_____

_____

_____

0 123456789 87

THIS COUPON ENTITLES YOU TO:

CREAM BLOWJOBS

0 123456789 87

TERMS & CONDITIONS:

_____

_____

_____

THIS COUPON ENTITLES YOU TO:

AN INTIMATE PICNIC

TERMS & CONDITIONS: _____

_____

_____

0 123456789 87

THIS COUPON ENTITLES YOU TO:

THREESOME

TERMS & CONDITIONS: _____

_____

_____

0 123456789 87

THIS COUPON ENTITLES YOU TO:

PORN MOVIE NIGHT

TERMS & CONDITIONS:

_____

_____

_____

0 123456789 87

THIS COUPON ENTITLES YOU TO:

WAKE-UP SEX

0 123456789 87

TERMS & CONDITIONS:

_____

_____

_____

THIS COUPON ENTITLES YOU TO:

YOUR DESIRED LINE OF DIRTY TALK DURING SEX

TERMS & CONDITIONS:

_____

_____

_____

0 123456789 87

THIS COUPON ENTITLES YOU TO:

BOOBJOB

TERMS & CONDITIONS:

_____

_____

_____

0 123456789 87

THIS COUPON ENTITLES YOU TO:

SIXTY-NINE

TERMS & CONDITIONS: _____

_____

_____

0 123456789 87

THIS COUPON ENTITLES YOU TO:

RIDE ME HARD

TERMS & CONDITIONS:
_____

_____

_____

0 123456789 87

THIS COUPON ENTITLES YOU TO:

ONE SPANKING SESSION

TERMS & CONDITIONS: _____

_____

_____

0 123456789 87

ONE ♥ PARKING SESSION

TERMS CONDITIONS

THIS COUPON ENTITLES YOU TO:

TAKE FULL CONTROL DURING SEX

TERMS & CONDITIONS: _____

_____

_____

0 123456789 87

THIS COUPON ENTITLES YOU TO:

ONE MUTUAL MASTURBATION SESSION

TERMS & CONDITIONS: _____

_____

_____

0 123456789 87

THIS COUPON ENTITLES YOU TO:

A NIGHT WITH BLINDFOLDS

0 123456789 87

TERMS & CONDITIONS:

_____

_____

_____

THIS COUPON ENTITLES YOU TO:

_____

TERMS & CONDITIONS: _____

_____

_____

0 123456789 87

THIS COUPON ENTITLES YOU TO:

0 123456789 87

TERMS & CONDITIONS:

THIS COUPON ENTITLES YOU TO:

0 123456789 87

TERMS & CONDITIONS:

THIS COUPON ENTITLES YOU TO:

_____

TERMS & CONDITIONS: _____

_____

_____

0 123456789 87

THIS COUPON ENTITLES YOU TO:

_____

0 123456789 87

TERMS & CONDITIONS: _____

_____

_____

THIS COUPON ENTITLES YOU TO:

TERMS & CONDITIONS:

0 123456789 87

THIS COUPON ENTITLES YOU TO:

_____

TERMS & CONDITIONS: _____

_____

_____

0 123456789 87

THIS COUPON ENTITLES YOU TO:

TERMS & CONDITIONS:

0 123456789 87

THIS COUPON ENTITLES YOU TO:

0 123456789 87

TERMS & CONDITIONS:

THIS COUPON ENTITLES YOU TO:

TERMS & CONDITIONS:

0 123456789 87

THANK YOU!

Thanks for buying *Sex Coupons For Him*.

If your found the book funny and enjoyed your time using the coupons, please share your thoughts about it on Amazon by leaving a review.

Also, if you want to discover more amazing books by Jackson Sweeters, check out his author page from Amazon. Just search "Jackson Sweeters" on Amazon's search bar and you'll find it.

Made in the USA
Monee, IL
22 September 2024

66304628R00070